QUICK ATKINS I

CW01500978

LOSE WEIGHT FAST WITH THESE 30 DELICIOUS 15-MINUTE MEALS

J.S. West

[FREE eBook LIMITED offer]

As a "Thank You" note to your interest in my recipe books, I'd like to offer my latest eBook for free up to 1000 amazon kindle downloads.
There aren't many left so grab your free copy now!

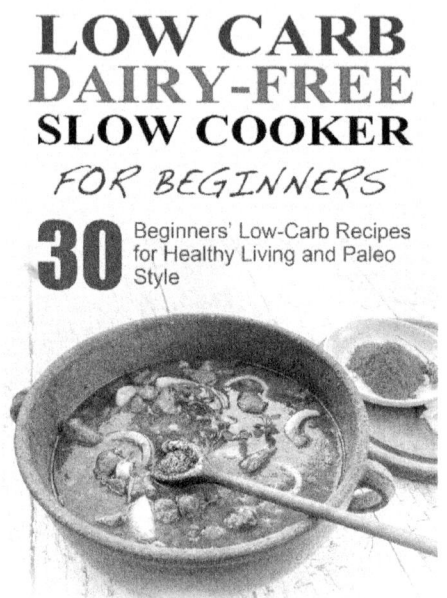

Click image to download

[JOIN FOR FREE]

presentation of the information is without contract or any type of guarantee assurance.

The trademarks that are used are without any consent, and the publication of the trademark is without permission or backing by the trademark owner. All trademarks and brands within this book are for clarifying purposes only and are the owned by the owners themselves, not affiliated with this document.

TABLE OF CONTENTS

INTRODUCTION

I want to thank you and congratulate you for downloading the book, "Quick Atkins Diet Recipes: Lose Weight Fast with These 30 Delicious 15-Minue Meals".

This book contains proven steps and strategies on how to transition into the Atkins diet and start losing weight fast. The sad truth is that over 50% of the American population is overweight and many don't know the first steps to losing that weight. With so many diet options available, it can be a bit overwhelming, but if you're reading this book that means you're interested in a lifestyle change.

This book will guide you through one of the most effective and easiest diet plans available. Throw away your calorie tracker and get rid of the "bad food" label for cheese and butter. Atkins is a highly effective diet regiment that allows you to shed the pounds fast and keep it off. It will take a good amount of self-control and motivation to stick to it since you'll be limiting your intake of carbohydrates. Once you see and feel the difference though, you'll never want to go back!

Thanks again for downloading this book, I hope you enjoy it!

CHAPTER 1 – WHAT IS ATKINS

Well before Robert Atkins came up with his namesake diet, versions of low carbohydrate diets have been around for centuries. In 1863 William Banting set England ablaze with a pamphlet that described a diet that gave up bread, butter, milk, sugar, beer and potatoes. In more modern times, Richard Mackarness published *Eat Fat and Grow Slim* back in 1958 that outlined the same basic theories that Robert Atkins later incorporated in his own theory. Finally, after several years of treating his own patients with low-carbohydrate diets, Robert Atkins published his *Dr. Atkins Diet Revolution* in 1972. While it met with some success, Atkins didn't reach the height of popularity until the late 1990s and early 2000s.

The Atkins diet follows a fairly simple theory. By limiting carb intake you force your body to burn stored fat instead of carbs for energy – a process called ketosis. According to Dr. Atkins extensive research and experimentation, the amount of calories and fat you consume don't affect your weight as strongly as your carbohydrate intake. So instead of tracking your calories, you will need to track your carb intake. Luckily, that's the only thing you need to limit. Atkins diet allows you to partake in almost all of your favorite foods and you don't need to feel guilty about it!

In order to really see the full benefit of Atkins, you'll need to follow the four phases:

Phase 1 - Induction: Probably the most difficult because this is where you have to severely limit your carb intake for your body to quickly enter the ketosis state. You'll need to limit your carbs to 20 grams per day for two weeks. All carbs consumed should only be low-carb, non-starchy vegetables like broccoli, leafy greens, pumpkin, tomatoes, turnips and asparagus. You should also consume 4 to 6 ounces of protein per meal, up to 4 ounces of cheese per day and 8 glasses of water. You should not eat any legumes, nuts or fruits in this phase. As well, you should not drink any alcohol in this stage.

Phase 2 – Ongoing Weight Loss

Once you've passed the two week hurdle of the induction phase, you can now slowly increase your carb intake by at 5 grams a week. The goal here is to find the "Critical Carbohydrate Level for Losing" and figure out what foods you can add in without triggering any carb cravings. Unlike the induction phase, this phase lasts until you are about 10 pounds away from your target weight. You can slowly being re-introducing some food groups back into your diet. For the first week of this phase you can add in some nuts and needs. After that you can include other foods weekly in the following order: berries, whole milk and yogurt.

Phase 3 – Pre-maintenance

In this phase, your weight loss will slow down as you increase your carb intake another 10 grams each week in order to find your "Critical Carbohydrate Level for Maintenance." Basically you're trying to find the maximum amount of carbs you can eat without gaining weight. You can start adding in things like legumes, some starchy vegetables and whole grains back into your diet once a week. Once you've finally reached your goal, you can adjust your carb intake by 10 grams each week and see if you gain weight or not. If you do gain weight you will need to cut back. It can take several weeks to find your individual tipping point, so don't get frustrated if you don't find your proper carb level immediately.

Phase 4 – Lifetime Maintenance

Once you have reached your goal weight and can maintain it without any fluctuations you are can move onto the last phase. Equipped with an arsenal of information, recipes and knowledge, you should be able to take your habits from previous phases and apply it to your everyday life.

Each phase will vary in length per the individual so don't be discouraged if you're not losing weight as fast as you think you should be. While Atkins certainly has the benefit of quick weight loss, especially in the beginning phase, it still takes dedication and motivation to stay on track and keep track of all of your carbs. Still, the positives outweigh the negatives. Studies have also shown that sustaining this diet increases your levels of HDL ("good" cholesterol), improves insulin resistance and lowers blood pressure. Weight loss research also suggests that those that follow the phases of Atkins properly are more likely to permanently keep off the weight they lost.

CHAPTER 2 – HEARTY INDUCTION MEALS

The induction phase might be the hardest on many people, but this is where you'll see the biggest weight loss results. Since your body can no longer rely on carbs for energy, it must use up the reserved fat that you've stored for its fuel. If done properly, you will easily see 5-10 pounds melt off. When paired with daily exercise the results will be even better!

Just because there aren't that many carbs in these two weeks doesn't mean that you can't enjoy a good meal. In fact, these recipes are so tasty you won't even miss the carbs! Below is a short list of items you can eat during the induction phase:

All fish

All poultry

All shellfish (mussels and oysters are high in carb so limit intake to 4 oz per day)

All meat (some processed meat like bacon and ham contain sugar, so limit your intake. Avoid cold cuts as they contain nitrates)

Eggs

Cheese: bleu, cheddar, goat cheese, cream cheese, feta cheese, gouda, mozzarella, parmesan and swiss

Very low-carb vegetables: alfalfa sprouts, arugula, bok choy, celery, chicory greens, chives, cucumber, endive, escarole, fennel, iceberg lettuce, mushrooms, parsley, peppers, radicchio, radishes, romaine lettuce,

Other suitable vegetables: artichoke, asparagus, avocados, broccoli, brussel sprouts, cabbage, cauliflower, swiss chard, collard greens, eggplant, green string beans, kale, kohlrabi, leeks, okra, onion, pumpkin, rhubarb, snow peas, spaghetti squash, spinach, tomato, turnips, zucchini

BREAKFAST

Herbed Asparagus Frittata

You will need:

6 large eggs

6 asparagus spears, chopped

4 tbs. of chopped chives

1 tbs. each of dried basil, parsley and oregano

1 tbs. butter

Salt and pepper to taste

Instructions

1. Preheat oven to broil.
2. Beat eggs in a medium mixing bowl and add in, chives, herbs and salt and pepper.
3. Melt butter in oven-safe skillet and add asparagus. Sauté for 2 to 3 minutes.
4. Pour egg mixture into pan and stir until evenly distributed.
5. Cook for about 4-5 minutes on medium-high heat or until eggs have set on the top and bottom.

6. Place pan into oven and broil for 3 to 4 minutes or until lightly brown. IMPORTANT: Be sure to keep an eye on the frittata as it will burn easily.
7. Once finished, remove frittata from pan and cut into servings. Serve immediately.

Eggs in a Basket

You will need:

4 eggs

4 slices of eggplant about 1" thick

1 tbs. extra virgin olive oil

1 tsp of butter

2 tsp of salt, divided

2 tsp of black pepper

2 tsp of dried rosemary, divided

Instructions

1. Preheat oven to broil
2. Brush the eggplants slices with olive oil and sprinkle with 1 tsp each of salt, pepper and rosemary.
3. Broil eggplants for approximately 3-4 minutes per side or until golden brown. Make sure to check in on your eggplants about 2 minutes in to make sure it doesn't burn.
4. Cut a hole in the center of each eggplant piece.
5. Melt butter in a large skillet and then place eggplants in it.

6. Crack egg into the center of the eggplant slice and season with remaining salt, rosemary and pepper.
7. Allow egg to cook for 3-4 minutes the flip.
8. Cook the other side for an additional 2-3 minutes until desired doneness is achieved.
9. Immediately take off pan and serve.

LUNCH

Chicken and asparagus salad

You will need:

1 chicken breast, sliced

3 asparagus spears, chopped

¼ cup of tomatoes, chopped

2 cups of romaine lettuce

1 tbs. extra virgin olive oil

1 tsp salt

1 tsp pepper

Salad dressing

2 tbs. apple cider vinegar

6 tbs. extra virgin olive oil

½ tsp salt

1 tsp pepper

1 tsp oregano

½ tsp rosemary

Instructions

1. Heat olive oil in a skillet on high heat. When properly heated, add sliced chicken and flavor with salt and pepper. Cook for about 3-5 minutes both sides, or until lightly browned. Add in chopped asparagus and cook around until tender, about 3-5 minutes.
2. Mix together the apple cider vinegar, salt, pepper, oregano and rosemary. Stir until salt dissolves. Whisk in the olive oil until fully incorporated.
3. Top romaine lettuce with the cooked chicken, asparagus and tomatoes.
4. Drizzle salad with dressing and serve.

Portobello Tuna Salad Sandwich

You will need:

2 large Portobello mushrooms, rinsed and de-stemmed

2 3 oz cans of tuna, drained

1 stalk of celery, diced

½ cup of raw alfalfa sprouts

2 tbs. of mayonnaise (Hellman's real mayonnaise)

1 tbs. of curry powder

1/2 tsp salt

1 tsp pepper

Instructions

1. In a skillet, lightly cook both sides of the Portobello mushroom caps for 2-3 minutes each side.
2. Combine the tuna, celery, mayonnaise, lemon juice, curry powder, salt and pepper in a medium mixing bowl. Mix until all ingredients are fully incorporated.
3. Top one mushroom cap with the tuna mixture and add alfalfa sprouts. Finish up by adding the last mushroom cap.

DINNER

Chili encrusted salmon with mashed cauliflower

You will need:

Salmon

½ lb of salmon

½ tbs chili powder

1 tsp cumin

½ tsp salt

¼ tsp pepper

Mashed Cauliflower

1 cup cauliflower florets

1 tbs. butter

1 glove of garlic, minced

¼ tsp salt

1/8 tsp pepper

Instructions

1. Preheat oven to 450 degrees F.
2. In a small mixing bowl combine chili powder, cumin and salt. Coat salmon well with mixture and place in baking dish skin down.
3. Roast for 10-12 minutes or until fish is flaky.
4. Meanwhile boil a large pot of water of high heat. Cook cut cauliflowers in boiling water until tender, about 10 minutes.
5. Drain well and pat the cauliflower dry.
6. Puree the hot cauliflower, garlic, butter, salt and pepper until almost smooth.
7. Plate the cauliflower mixture and top with salmon. Include lemon wedges if desired.

Cheesy Spinach Chicken with Arugula Salad

You will need:

Chicken

4-5 thinly sliced skinless, boneless chicken tenders

1 cup of spinach, rinsed

2 ounces of mozzarella cheese, shredded

1 tbs. butter

1 tbs. olive oil

2 tsp of salt, divided

1 tsp of pepper, divided

1 glove of garlic, minced

Toothpicks

Arugula Salad

> 1 cup arugula

> 3 raw radishes, thinly sliced

> Apple cider vinegar dressing

Instructions

1. Melt butter in medium skillet over high heat. Add in garlic and sauté until garlic for 3-5 minutes or until lightly browned. Add in spinach and cook for another 3 minutes until wilted. Season with 1 tsp of salt and ½ tsp of pepper.
2. Divide spinach mixture and cheese evenly to the chicken tenders and roll up. Sprinkle salt and pepper evenly over the stuffed chicken. Secure with toothpick.
3. Heat olive oil in skillet then add rolled chicken to the pan. Cook until browned on both sides, about 5 minutes each.
4. Remove chicken from pan and fan serve on dinner plate. Add arugula and radish to the plate and drizzle with apple cider vinegar dressing.

SNACK

Deviled eggs

You will need:

> 6 eggs

> ¼ cup mayonnaise (Hellman's real mayonnaise)

> 1 tsp. yellow mustard

1 tsp. white wine vinegar

Salt and pepper to taste

Paprika (optional)

Instructions

1. Place eggs in a large sauce pan and cover with water.
2. Heat on high and bring water to a rolling boil. Continue boiling for a minute, then turn off the heat and cover the pan with a fitted lid. Let sit for 10 minutes.
3. Immediately cool the eggs down with ice cold water and peel. Slice the peeled eggs length wise and pop out the eggs yolks into a fine mesh sieve. Set the sieve over a medium sized bowls and push the egg yolks through.
4. Mix in the mayonnaise, mustard, vinegar and salt and pepper to the mashed yolks and mix until well incorporated. Adjust seasonings to taste.
5. Spoon egg mixture back into the egg whites.

Chapter 3 – Flavorful OWL Recipes

Now that your body has undergone ketosis, you can begin increasing the amount of carbs you consume by 5 grams per day. What's better is that you can start adding back in nuts and seeds, berries and heavy milk products back into your diet. Keep track of the amount of weight you are losing. If you're weight loss has plateaued, cut back on your carb intake again. There's no set time limit for the ongoing weight loss (OWL) phase so you'll also need to practice some patience as you are likely to see slight weight fluctuations as you adjust your carbs. Keep working at this phase until you are 10 pounds away from your target weight.

After going without for the past two weeks, you're sure to appreciate the added food groups even more.

BREAKFAST

Tofu Pesto Scramble

You will need:

Tofu

> 1 14-ounce blocks of extra firm tofu, crumbled
>
> 1 ½ tsp. turmeric
>
> 1 garlic clove, minced
>
> 2 ounces mozzarella cheese, grated
>
> 1 tbs. butter

Pesto

1 cup fresh basil

¼ cup sunflower seeds

1 tbs. lemon juice

1 tbs. extra virgin olive oil

Instructions

1. In a blender, combine all of the ingredients for the pesto and blend until smooth. Set aside.
2. Drain water from the tofu backs and dry excess water on paper towels. Finely crumble tofu in a medium sized bowl.
3. Over high heat melt the butter then add the garlic. Sauté until garlic is lightly browned, about 5 minutes. Add crumbled tofu and turmeric and cook for 2-3 minutes.
4. Add in cheese and cook for an additional 2-3 minutes until cheese is fully melted.
5. Plate the tofu scramble and top with pesto.

Pork Rind Pancakes

You will need:

4 eggs

1/2 cup heavy cream

3 oz bag of unflavored pork rinds

1 tsp pure vanilla extract

Cinnamon and nutmeg to taste

1 tbs. butter.

¼ cup of raspberries

Instructions

1. Crumble pork rinds into a medium bowl until they look like breadcrumbs.
2. In a separate bowl, beat eggs until frothy, then add in all the other ingredients except the pork rinds. Continue beating until well mixed.
3. Add in the pork rinds and let it site for 5 minutes until batter thickens.
4. Melt butter in a skillet over high heat. Spoon half of the batter onto the skillet. Cook both sides until lightly browned, about 3-5 minutes on each side.
5. Remove immediately from heat and serve with ¼ cup of fresh raspberries.

LUNCH

Crunchy Kale and Shrimp Salad

You will need:

1 cup of kale, chopped with stems removed

6 large shrimps, de-shelled and de-veined

1/8 cup of cherry tomatoes, halved

7 walnut halves, chopped

2 tbs. extra virgin olive oil, separated

Salt and pepper to taste

Strawberry vinaigrette dressing

¼ cup sliced strawberries

¼ cup of extra virgin olive oil

1 tsp whole grain mustard

2 tbs. red wine vinegar

1 packet of Splenda

Salt and pepper to taste

Instructions

1. Puree strawberries in a blender until smooth. Add in the vinegar, mustard and seasonings. Blend until incorporated. Add in olive oil and blend until creamy. Adjust seasonings to taste. Pour into a small container and set aside.
2. Preheat oven to 350 degrees F.
3. In a large mixing bowl add kale, sale and olive. Toss the kale until all leaves are coated evenly.
4. Place kale on a baking tray in a single layer and bake until edges are browned, about 10 to 15 minutes.
5. While the kale is baking, heat up the remaining olive oil in a skillet over high heat. Add the shrimp and season with salt and pepper. Cook until both sides have turned pink and form a "C" shape, about 2 minutes on both sides.
6. Combine the shrimp, kale, tomatoes and walnuts into a salad bowl and drizzle with strawberry vinaigrette.

Thai Chicken and Zucchini Noodles

You will need:

Chicken and Noodles

½ lb. of chicken, sliced

1 ½ cups of zucchini, shredded or spiralized

½ cup of red cabbage, finely shredded

1 tsp olive oil

Salt and pepper to taste

Peanut sauce dressing

1 tbs. natural peanut butter

½ tbs. of water

½ tbs. apple cider vinegar

½ tbs. Tamari

1 garlic clove minced

½ tsp. sesame oil

½ tsp. ginger, grated

Instructions

1. Place the zucchini noodles and cabbage in a paper towel lined serving bowl. Set aside.
2. Heat sesame oil in a skillet over high heat. Add in chicken and season with salt and pepper. Cook until both sides are browned, about 5 minutes each side. Remove from heat.
3. In a small bowl, whisk together the peanut butter, water and remaining ingredients. If it is too difficult to mix, add in extra water making sure that the sauce does not become too runny.

4. Remove paper towels from under the zucchini noodles and add in the cooked chicken. Add the peanut sauce and stir until the noodles, chicken and cabbage are evenly coated with sauce.

DINNER

Seared Shrimp with Bacon-y Brussel Sprouts

You will need:

Shrimp

> 6 large shrimp
>
> 1 tbs. olive oil, divided
>
> Salt and pepper to taste

Brussel Sprouts

> 1 cup of brussel sprouts, shredded
>
> 1 shallot, thinly sliced
>
> 2 strips of bacon
>
> Salt and pepper to taste

Instructions

1. Heat a skillet over medium-high heat and add bacon. Cook on both sides until most of the fat is rendered and the bacon begins to crisp, about 2-3 minutes.
2. Add in brussel sprouts and shallots and season with salt and pepper. Cook until the shallots are browned, about 5 minutes.

3. Transfer to a plate and set aside. Wipe off excess oil from skillet.
4. Pat shrimp dry with a paper towel and season with salt and pepper.
5. Heat oil in skillet over high heat. Add shrimp and sear on both sides for 2-3 minutes.
6. Serve shrimp over the brussel sprouts.

Chicken Stir-fry

½ lb. boneless, skinless chicken breast, sliced

1/2 cup baby bok choy, washed

1 8 oz. can bamboo shoots

½ cup snow peas

1 tbs. Tamari

1 tbs. peanut oil

Salt and pepper to taste

Instructions

1. Heat peanut oil in wok over high heat. Add chicken breast and cook for 5-6 minutes.
2. Add in vegetables, soy sauce, salt and pepper. Cook until the vegetables are soft, about 5 minutes.

SNACKS

Butter roasted pecans

You will need:

20 pecan halves

1 tbs. of butter, melted

¼ tsp of sea salt

Instructions

1. Preheat the oven to 350 degrees F.
2. Toss together the pecans and melted butter in a medium bowl.
3. Spread pecans in a single layer on a baking sheet and sprinkle sea salt over them.
4. Bake until fragrant, about 15 minutes. Remove from heat and let cool.

Kohlrabi Fries

You will need:

1 kohlrabi, peeled

½ tsp salt

1/8 tsp pepper

¼ tsp. cumin

Cayenne pepper to taste

4 tbs. of olive oil

Instructions

1. Combine spices in a small bowl and set aside.
2. Heat the oil in a heavy skillet over medium-high heat.
3. Meanwhile, slice kohlrabi length-wise into thirds, then cut into ¼ inch slices.
4. When the oil starts rippling add in the kohlrabi sticks to the pan in batches. Cook each side until browned, about

2-3 minutes. Remove from oil and drain on paper towers. Season with spice mixture and serve.

CHAPTER 4 – DROOLWORTHY PRE-MAINTENANCE RECIPES

Congratulations! You've made it Phase 3. It doesn't matter how long it took you to get here, what matters is that you finally arrived to the penultimate step. If you properly made your way through Phase 2, this means that you are now within 10 pounds of your ideal weight. You'll be losing weight at a much slower pace, but that's the idea. This phase is all about fine-tuning your carb intake until you will find your personal carb balance or Atkins Carbohydrate Equilibrium (ACE). You'll add even more variety to your diet by adding starchy vegetables, legumes and whole grains in small 10 additional grams of carbs a week. Not only are you seeing how much carbs you can add back in but what types of carbs as well. You may have a high tolerance and find that you can eat all of these food items or you might need to forego some of them.

You can easily up your carb intake by eating one of these fruits a week: apple, banana, cherry, grapefruit, guava, kiwi, mango, peach, plum and watermelon. They serve as a great snack and will help curb your sugar cravings.

Of course, you can add in the additional carbs to your daily meals as well. Now that you have free reign over grains and legumes, your options are practically endless!

BREAKFAST

Carrot Pancakes

You will need:

1 carrot, grated

½ cup pecans

¼ cup water

2 eggs

1 packet of Splenda

¼ tsp baking powder

Cinnamon and nutmeg to taste

Pinch of salt

Instructions

1. Grind pecans in a food processor. Add spices, salt and baking powder and pulse until well blended. Transfer to a medium sized bowl.
2. Combine the wet ingredients in another bowl and mix well. Add in the dry ingredients and mix until batter is combined.
3. Heat skillet over medium heat and spoon ¼ cup into the skillet. Cook until browned on both sides, about 3-5 minutes.

No Bake Chocolate Banana Muffins

You will need:

¼ cup of ground flax seeds

1 egg

2 tsp unsweetened cocoa

½ of a ripe banana

1 ½ packets of Splenda

Instructions

1. Blend ingredients together until combined.
2. Pour batter into a cup and microwave on high for 1-2 minutes.
3. Allow to cool for 5 minutes then serve.

LUNCH

Salmon Stuffed Avocado

You will need:

1 ripe avocado

½ cup of cucumber, chopped

1 cup smoked salmon, chopped

¼ cup canned chick peas

1 tsp. lemon juice

1 tsp. dill

Salt and pepper to taste

Instructions

1. Cut avocado in half length-wise and remove the stone.
2. Gently scoop out the insides, taking care not to break the skin's shell.
3. In a bowl mash the avocado flesh then combine salmon, chick peas, lemon juice, dill and salt and pepper.
4. Fill the avocado shells and serve.

Chopped Apple and Chicken Salad *(16.4 grams of carbs)*

You will need:

> ½ cup of chicken, chopped
>
> 4 cups romaine lettuce
>
> ½ of an apple, chopped
>
> ¼ tomato, chopped
>
> 2 tbs. crumbled bleu cheese
>
> ½ an avocado, chopped
>
> 1 tbs. olive oil
>
> Apple cider vinegar vinaigrette

Instructions

1. Heat oil in a skillet over high heat. Add in chicken and cook until done about 10 minutes.
2. In a large salad bowl, combine lettuce, apple, tomato, chicken, avocado and bleu cheese. Top with vinaigrette and toss until all ingredients are evenly distributed.

DINNER

Citrus Turkey Burger in Lettuce "Buns"

You will need:

> ½ lb. of ground turkey
>
> 1 tsp. grated grapefruit rind

2 tsp. grapefruit juice

¼ tsp. dried basil

¼ tsp. dried oregano

Salt and pepper to taste

2 cups Iceberg lettuce leaves

1 tbs. mayonnaise

Tomato slices

Instructions

1. Combine all ingredients except the mayonnaise and iceberg lettuce into a large mixing bowl. Once all ingredients are mixed well, form into burger patties.
2. Grill on both sides until done, about 5-10 minutes on both sides. If you do not have a grill, cook in a skillet over medium-high heat for 7-10 minutes, or until done.
3. Assemble the turkey burger and additional burger toppings in the lettuce leaves.

Roasted Cod with Butter with Garlic Lentils

You will need:

Cod

7 oz. of skinless cod fillets

1 tbs. butter, softened

1 garlic glove, minced

1 tsp. lemon juice

1/8 tsp. Dijon mustard

1 tbs. chopped prosciutto

1 tsp. almond flour

1 tbs. olive oil

Salt and pepper to taste

Lemon wedge for garnish

Lentils

¼ cup of lentils, washed

1 tbs. butter

2 garlic glove, minced

Salt and pepper to taste

Instructions

1. In a medium pot, add lentils and ¾ cup of water. Bring water to a soft simmer and cook uncovered for about 15-20 minutes.
2. Meanwhile stir together butter, garlic, lemon juice, mustard, almond flour, prosciutto, salt and pepper in a small bowl and set aside.
3. Preheat oven to 450 degrees F.
4. When lentils are almost done, heat the oil in an oven-proof skillet over medium-high heat. Season cod fillets with salt and pepper and cook in skillet on one side for 4 minutes. Turn and cook for an additional 1 minute.
5. Spoon butter mixture over fillets and bake in oven for 2 minutes or until fish is cooked through.
6. Melt butter in skillet over high heat. Add garlic and cook until browned, about 5 minutes. Add in lentils and

sauté for 1 minute. Plate lentils and top with cod. Pour any additional sauce from the fish skillet over the top.

SNACKS

Cauli-Tots

You will need:

1 12 oz bag of frozen cauliflower

3 oz. of Parmesan cheese, grated

Salt, pepper and garlic powder to taste

Instructions

1. Preheat oven to 400 degrees F.
2. Microwave cauliflower for 6 minutes on high heat. Pour off water and cool.
3. Process in a food processor until smooth.
4. Meanwhile combine Parmesan cheese with garlic powder, salt and pepper in a small bowl.
5. Shape pureed cauliflower into 1.5" balls while squeezing out excess water then drop into Parmesan mixture.
6. Place cauli-tots on a baking sheet and bake for 10 minutes.

Cherry Cheesecake

You will need:

Cheesecake

2 oz of cream cheese, softened

1 egg

1 tbs. Splenda

1 tsp. lemon juice

½ tsp. pure vanilla extract

Cherry topping

¼ cup frozen cherries

1 tbs. Splenda

3 tbs. water

½ tsp. pure vanilla extract

Instructions

Cherry Topping

1. Thaw cherries in microwave for 3 minutes.
2. Combine cherries, Splenda and water in a medium saucepan. Bring mixture to a boil then reduce heat to simmer.
3. Add in vanilla and simmer until sauce thickens, about 10-15 minutes

Cheesecake

1. Mix together softened cream cheese and egg in a microwave safe cup or small bowl until well incorporated.
2. Add in the remaining ingredients.
3. Microwave on high for 2 minutes.
4. Top with cherry sauce

Chapter 5 – Wholesome Life Maintenance Meals

Before you look at the recipes, give yourself a pat on the back. You've finally made it! The final phase isn't really a phase per se; it's more of a permanent lifestyle. You will take all that you've learned from the previous steps and apply them to your everyday eating habits. At this point you should know what starchy vegetables, fruits and whole grains you can consume and what you cannot to maintain your weight. You might also need to make adjustments as you grow through various life changes, but luckily after completing all of the previous phases, you'll know exactly what to do.

The foods you can eat in this phase are the same ones from Phase 3 so there shouldn't be any drastic changes to your diet. You can continue re-introducing some foods that you did not in Phase 3 so long as you are alert to what foods cause weight regain and cravings for you.

With this final phase, you can finally say goodbye to on-again, off-again diets.

BREAKFAST

Breakfast Bacon Sandwich

You will need:

> 1 tbs. butter, separated
>
> 4 slices of bacon

¼ cup water

2 large eggs

Salt and pepper to taste

Biscuit cutter

Instructions

1. Heat a skillet over low heat. Add the 4 slices of bacon and cook until browned evenly on both sides, about 5-7 minutes each side.
2. Remove from heat and drain on a paper towel. Pour off excess bacon grease into a cup.
3. Crack each egg into a separate small bowl. Pierce the yolks with a fork.
4. Use ½ tbs. of butter to grease the inside of the biscuit cutter.
5. Melt the remaining butter in a skillet over medium high heat. Place the biscuit cutters in the pan and then pour the egg into each mold.
6. Season the eggs with salt and pepper.
7. Add the water to the skillet (outside of the egg molds) and cover. Cook for 3 minutes or until cooked through.
8. To serve, separate the eggs from the egg molds. Sandwich the bacon between the two egg ends.

Strawberry Crepes

You will need:

Crepe

2 eggs

2.5 oz. cream cheese

½ tsp cinnamon

½ tbs. Splenda

1 tbs. butter

Filling

¼ Frozen strawberries

2 tbs. butter

1 tbs. Splenda

Instructions

1. Blend all crepe ingredients (except butter) in a blender until smooth.
2. Let batter rest for 5 minutes.
3. Melt butter in a skillet over medium heat then add enough batter in the skillet to form a 6-inch crepe. Cook for about 2 minutes then flip and cook for an additional minute. Remove to plate. Repeat until all batter is used.
4. Meanwhile thaw strawberries in microwave in high heat for 3-4 minutes.
5. In a medium saucepan, melt butter over high heat then add strawberries and Splenda. Cook for 3-5 minutes.
6. To serve, spread 1 tbs. of mixture into the center of your crepes. Roll up and sprinkle with additional Splenda if desired.

LUNCH

Bacon and Apple Melt

You will need:

1 apple, sliced ½"thick

4-6 slices of bacon

2 oz mozzarella cheese, grated

1 tbs. basil, chopped

Instructions

1. Preheat toaster oven to 350 degrees F.
2. Heat a skillet over low heat. Add the 4 slices of bacon and cook until browned evenly on both sides, about 5-7 minutes each side.
3. Remove from heat and drain on a paper towel. Pour off excess bacon grease into a cup.
4. Layer as follows: apple slice, bacon, basil, apple slice and top with cheese. Repeat for additional sandwiches.
5. Bake in toaster oven until cheese is melted, about 5-10 minutes.

Smoked Salmon and Avocado Roll-up

You will need

¼ cup brown rice, cooked

1 avocado, pitted and thinly sliced

½ cucumber, halved and sliced

6 slices of smoked salmon

Instructions

1. For each smoked salmon, place a small amount of rice and a couple avocado and cucumber slices. Roll up salmon to enclose rich and avocado.
2. Secure with toothpicks and serve.

DINNER

Zucchini Crab Cakes

You will need:

 3 zucchinis, grated

 ½ container of extra firm tofu, drained and crumbled

 1 can of crab meat, drained

 1 tbs. Old Bay seasoning

 1 tbs. olive oil

 Lemon wedge garnish

Instructions

1. In a medium mixing bowl, combine zucchini, tofu, crab meat and old bay seasoning. Mix until well combined.
2. Form zucchini-crab mixture into 3 inch patties.
3. Heat olive oil in a skillet over high heat. Add patties into skillet. Cook until both sides are browned, about 3-5 minutes.
4. Top with additional Old Bay seasoning if necessary and serve with a wedge of lemon. *Suggested Sides: Mashed cauliflower, kohlrabi fries.*

Peachy Pork Chops

You will need:

 2 bone-in pork chops

 1 fresh peach, sliced

1 tbs. water

1 tbs. Splenda

1 tbs. balsamic vinegar

1 tbs. olive oil

1 tsp. garlic powder

½ tsp. chili powder

Salt and pepper to taste

Instructions

1. Season pork chops evenly with garlic powder, chili powder and salt and pepper.
2. Heat oil in large skillet on medium heat. Add pork chops and cook 4 minutes per side or until desired doneness. Remove from skillet; keep warm.
3. Add water, sugar and vinegar to the same skillet and bring to a boil. Add in peaches and simmer for 2 minutes. Spoon over pork chops and serve. *Suggested sides: Cauli-tots, arugula salad.*

SNACKS

Guacamole

You will need:

1 avocado, pitted

1 tbs. lime juice

1 tbs. cilantro, chopped

1 plum tomato, chopped

1 small garlic clove, minced

Salt and pepper to taste

Instructions

1. In a medium bowl, mash together the avocados, lime juice and salt until smooth.
2. Mix in the cilantro, garlic and tomatoes. Serve immediately with baby carrots, broccoli and cauliflower or refrigerate.

Chilled Watermelon Soup

You will need:

1 cup watermelon, cubed and seeded

½ tsp of lemon juice

1 tsp. freshly chopped mint

½ tsp of Splenda

¼ tsp grated ginger

¾ cup plain nonfat yogurt

Mint sprigs for garnish

Instructions

1. Blend all ingredients in a blender until smooth.
2. Cool for 15 minutes in a freezer or refrigerate for 2 hours for best results.
3. Garnish with mint sprigs before serving.

CONCLUSION

Thank you again for downloading this book!

I hope this book was able to help give you the information and recipes you need to jumpstart your Atkins diet. As you can see from these recipes, there is no shortage of flavor when on this diet nor will you ever have to feel hungry throughout the day. As with any diets, be sure to consult with your primary physician before making any changes.

The next step is to commit use these recipes as a base guideline and get creative. You can experiment with a number of different flavors to suit your needs. Happy eating!

OTHER RECOMMENDED BOOKS

<u>Paleo for Beginners: Essentials to Get Started with the Paleo Diet</u> (Click to on title go to Amazon link)

Book Description

The Paleo diet is not just another fad diet; it is the diet humans were designed to eat. Also known as the Primal diet, the Caveman diet, and the Stone Age diet, the Paleo diet focuses on low-carb, high-protein meals, and removes all processed foods.

Paleo for Beginners will show you how to adopt a Paleo lifestyle in order to feel healthy, lose weight, and increase your energy level. With Paleo for Beginners, start enjoying the best health of your life today--all while losing weight and decreasing your odds of diabetes, hypertension, heart disease, cancer, osteoporosis, and many other modern health maladies.

This is A Preview Of What You'll Learn...

Successfully make the transition to a Paleo lifestyle with a 7-day, step-by-step plan for beginners

Set yourself up for success with the Paleo shopping guide and a list of 117 Paleo-recommended foods (and an extensive list of what food items you should avoid).

Enjoy Paleo-friendly versions of 99 mouthwatering recipes for every meal. Recipes include Eggs Benedict Paleo Style, High-Protein Grain-Free Burgers, Chicken Avocado Wraps, and Paleo Waffles.

OTHER BOOKS FROM J.S. WEST

Amazon
Kindle

Click Images
for Links

go to
J.S. West
Author Page

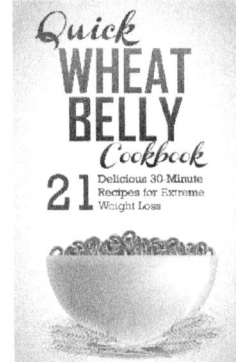

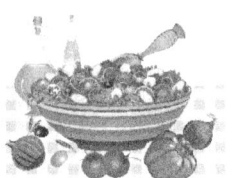

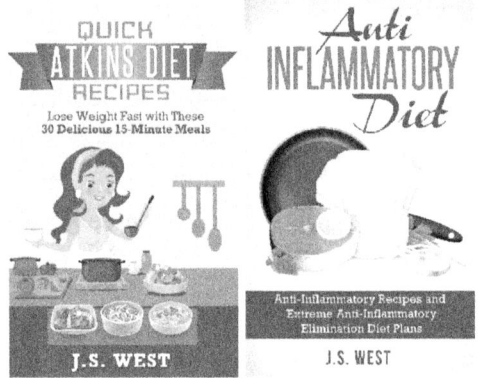

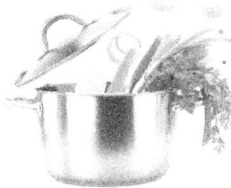

LOW CARB CROCK POT
Cookbook

25 Quick and Easy Slow Cooker Paleo Diet Recipes for Busy People to Lose Weight Fast

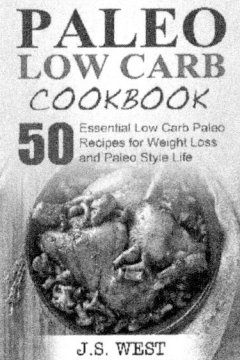

PALEO LOW CARB COOKBOOK

50 Essential Low Carb Paleo Recipes for Weight Loss and Paleo Style Life

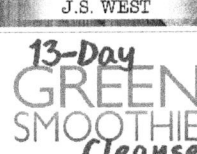

J.S. WEST

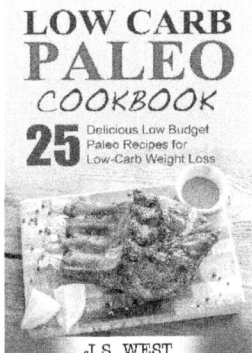

LOW CARB PALEO COOKBOOK

25 Delicious Low Budget Paleo Recipes for Low-Carb Weight Loss

J.S. WEST

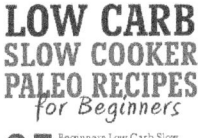

LOW CARB SLOW COOKER PALEO RECIPES *for Beginners*

25 Beginners Low Carb Slow Cooker Recipes for Extreme Weight Loss and Paleo Style

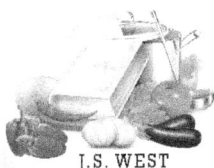

J.S. WEST

13-Day GREEN SMOOTHIE *Cleanse*

Extreme Weight Loss and Paleo Style

J.S. WEST

Amazon
Kindle

Click Images for Links

go to
J.S. West
Author Page

OTHER BOOKS FROM J.S. WEST

<u>Paleo Diet: Paleo Low Carb Slow Cooker Recipes for Beginners - Weight Loss and Paleo Style</u> (Click to on title go to Amazon link)

Book Description

Many people in today's society are unhappy with the state of their health and wellbeing. Some want to lose weight; others have frequent stomach upset that interferes with daily life. Still others have skin problems or emotional irritability that can be easily related to eating foods that are not healthy for the body.

Early man did not have these kinds of problems. "Cavemen," as most people refer to them, ate what they could hunt, find, and pluck from the trees. They were fit and not overweight, and were generally quite healthy. The paleo diet is a recent lifestyle based on the overall food consumption of the early man, and the trend is quickly gaining popularity. It has many proven and documented health benefits, including weight loss, improved digestive systems, and increased energy levels without the use of caffeine.

This book should serve as a helpful resource for anyone looking to get started on a paleo diet. The first part of the book will explain, briefly, the definition of a paleo diet, what can and cannot be eaten when following a paleo diet, and the items most necessary to keep in stock in a paleo-friendly kitchen. The rest of the book will be devoted to paleo recipes that can be cooked either completely or almost completely in a slow cooker. These recipes will be simple, but tasty, and will be perfect options for those who are just beginning to learn about paleo dieting. A slow cooker is a very easy and affordable option for cooking new recipes and starting a new diet, since the food can be prepared ahead of time and kept warm safely for hours.

This is A Preview Of What You'll Learn...

You will be excited and ready to try eating "like a caveman" in your own life. The health and wellness benefits will be incredible!

an understanding of the paleo diet and its benefits

what ingredients you need to set up a paleo kitchen

easy and delicious paleo slow cooker recipes

sample paleo meal plans

and much, much more!

[JOIN FOR FREE]

If you liked this book I'm sure that YOU will LIKE my other books as well.

Join my mailing list and get updates on FREE deals, new releases, bonus content and many others.

Click Here To Sign Up

THANK YOU!!

Thank you again for downloading our book!

I hope this book was able to help you to achieve your health goals.

The next step is to apply what you've learned in this book and try out the great recipes provided.

If you enjoyed this book, please share your thoughts and leave a review on Amazon. Your feedback is important to us in order to improve the quality of the book.

CLICK HERE to LEAVE REVIEW

Good luck!

Printed in Great Britain
by Amazon

47437148R00030